Raw Vegan Food Is A Better Life For Me

An Interesting Story of Love for Raw Vegan Food. Why to Choose Raw Vegan Food? How to Get Rid of Diseases to Be Young, Beautiful and Successful.

Foreword

The first time my friend told me about a raw vegan diet, I was really confused since I could not imagine my days without heavy meals.

Her story was quite inspiring, though. After years of struggling with allergies, low energy, and problems with digestive system, my friend and her husband decided to make some positive changes to improve their lives. They used to enjoy heavy meals not realizing that this was the actual cause of their state.

So, they gradually turned to a raw food diet, and they first noticed that they felt happier and full of energy. Because of this, they decided that a raw vegan diet should be a part of their lifestyle. Now, their two little daughters also enjoy a variety of raw food and are simply bursting with life.

Her story inspired me to learn more about raw food and its benefits. I've collected information from a variety of sources – books, interviews with doctors, nutrition experts as well as raw vegans and their experiences with this kind of diet. As I have witnessed how raw food can bring positive changes to one's life, I thought that it is time to spread the word about this.

I would like to thank my friend for inspiring me to write this book. *Raw Vegan Food Is a Better Life for Me* is my way to show how grateful I am to her for sharing her story with me. This is the first one in a series of books I'm planning to publish on this topic. I sincerely hope that you too will discover the vibrancy that raw food can bring to our lives.

Table of Contents

Introduction

When you think of raw food diet, you probably think how vibrant, colorful, pure and bursting with life it is. It provides you with a way to give your body a whole variety of dense nutrients.

There is a belief that when food is processed, its nutrients get destroyed and your body gets almost nothing from it. In that sense, raw food diet is based on the idea that your body will stay healthy if you consume food in its natural form, as this kind of diet will help you avoid all sorts of diseases. What is even more, if you are concerned with your weight, you can be sure that you will manage to lose some pounds since this diet is mostly high in fiber and low in fat and calories. However, you should also bear in mind that you should provide your body with enough protein, calcium, iron and some vitamins because you will have to avoid animal products. Although this is a raw food diet, it doesn't mean that cooking is that bad. For instance, cooking has its benefits as well such as killing bacteria and boosting some nutrients. So, you can make use of this and eat some steamed vegetables from time to time.

As you can assume, this kind of diet allows you to enjoy a whole variety of vegetables, fruits, grains, nuts and seeds, and when preparing your meals, you can use food processors, blenders, and dehydrators. You may think that having various cookbooks and getting all the necessary kitchen utensils is enough for following this diet properly. However, you, as a newbie, are still likely to make some mistakes. Hopefully for you, besides various tips on a raw food diet, this book will also help you avoid some common mistakes.

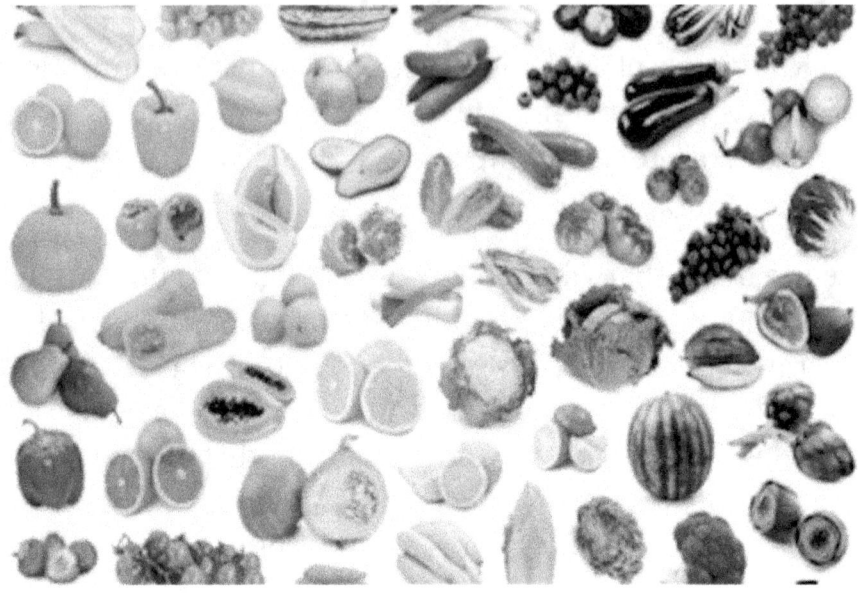

You will need to put in some extra effort to prepare your meals because you may have to walk from one grocery to another or even find some specialty stores to find organic and healthy foods. Don't get scared now. You will eventually realize that this will do a world of good for your health. This diet works well both for vegans and vegetarians but in any case you should make sure that this diet meets the needs of your body.

If you are still positive about going raw, read on to discover some guidelines and tips on how to make raw foods part of your routine.

Chapter 1: What is processed food and why is it bad for us?

Any alteration to food as it is normally found may be called processing. Cooking in any form like boiling, frying, microwaving, barbecuing, etc. can also be called processing. Since additives are added when foods are canned, canning and preserving food in any form for long periods is also a form of processing. So, it appears almost impossible to avoid this kind of food.

Many processed packed foods like cookies, breads, noodles, etc. usually contain huge amounts of sugar, salt, high fructose corn syrup or HFCS, MSG and other harmful additives. HFCS alone is enough to wreck one's health. In fact, the 'apparently harmless' refined sugar is known to be more addictive than cocaine! If you don't trust me, just try to eliminate refined sugar from your diet altogether, and you will understand what I mean. High levels of sugar and salt in our normal diets bring a lot of problems with them. This kind of diet on a sustained basis is responsible for many adverse impacts on our bodies. One thing it does is elevating insulin levels in our bodies, and this ultimately leads to insulin resistance.

Unfortunately, the standard diet in the developed world is such that we are exposed to these harmful substances on a regular basis, day in and day out. Diabetes and high blood sugar have taken the form of an epidemic in the developed world. Cholesterol is another by-product of this type of diet, the consequence of which is widespread heart-related conditions that are becoming very common nowadays and have started affecting younger people as well. This kind of diet also brings with it carcinogenic substances, and cancer is the next big epidemic about to happen. Strangely, the major sufferers from these types of "lifestyle diseases" (I hope you understand why they are called like this) are people from the developed world, and people from the traditionally poorer countries are not yet affected by these in a big way.

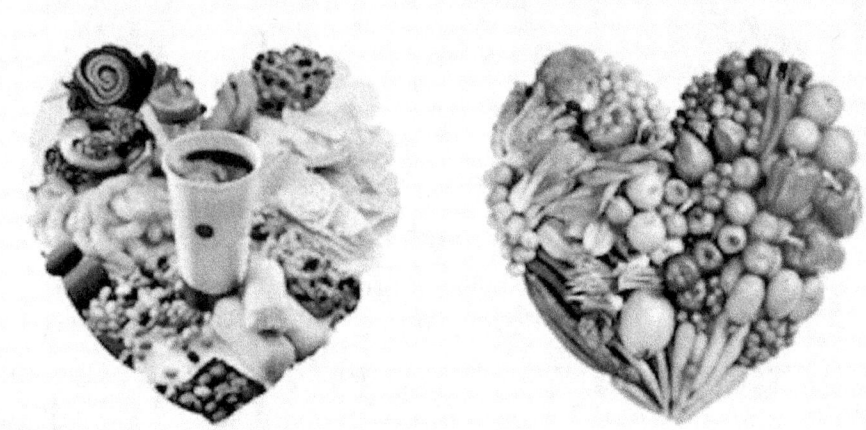

What does cooking do to our food?

When anything is cooked (fried or baked or just heated), it goes through Maillard reaction. Maillard reaction is defined as "a chemical reaction between amino acids and reducing sugars that gives browned foods their colour and the desirable flavour". So, you may conclude that boiled foods are unaffected by it.

Maillard reaction releases advanced glycation end-products (AGEs) into our bodies. In an effort to make food tasty and digestible, we are doing ourselves more harm than good. AGE's are major oxidants. It means they are responsible for the aging process of the body and are to bodies what rust is to a machine. In other words, they make our bodies age faster.

The body reacts to AGE's as if it were an infection. In fact, after you eat cooked food, the white blood cells, the infection fighters of our body, rush to our digestive system thinking it to be an infection, thus leaving the rest of our system unprotected and susceptible to a disease break-in. This phenomenon is called "digestive leukocytosis".

In 1930, the Swiss researchers at the institute of Chemical Chemistry found that eating raw, unaltered food did not cause "digestive leukocytosis". They found that this happened only when food had been heated beyond a certain temperature which is unique to each food. This also happened in cases in which the food was processed or refined or chemicals were added to it. It is clear that digestive leukocytosis is a result of cooked food.

Food affected by Maillard-reaction also have a tendency to stick to our arteries, thus causing blockage, heart trouble and high blood pressure, skin inflammations, obesity and insulin resistance. In fact, cooked food pushes us towards obesity. Since cooked food fails to supply cells with enough nutrients, they are always hungry for more, and this promotes overeating in a lot of us and thus leads to obesity.

Eating cooked food leads to accumulation of toxins in our bodies, and getting rid of these puts a lot of pressure on our bodies. Our headaches, nausea, fever, colds, vomiting, sinusitis, bronchitis, pneumonia, diarrhea, and other such symptoms originate from an overworked digestive system.

The RAW FOOD Pyramid

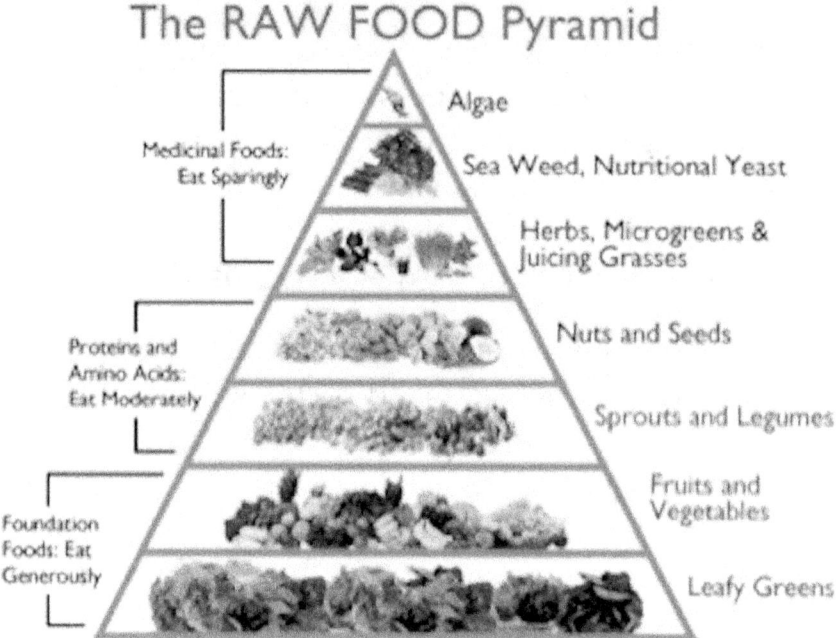

Medicinal Foods: Eat Sparingly

- Algae
- Sea Weed, Nutritional Yeast
- Herbs, Microgreens & Juicing Grasses

Proteins and Amino Acids: Eat Moderately

- Nuts and Seeds
- Sprouts and Legumes

Foundation Foods: Eat Generously

- Fruits and Vegetables
- Leafy Greens

Let us see what else happens to food when we cook it:

- The nutrient makeup and biomechanical structure of the food are degraded, deranged, and broken down, rendering the food less effective.
- Amino acids, nutrients, and vitamins are either destroyed or altered.
- Almost 50% of the protein gets coagulated, rendering it useless for us.
- A jump in the numbers of cancer-causing free radicals is noticed after cooking.
- The food gets dehydrated.
- Digesting cooked food takes much more energy than digesting raw food.
- Intestines get clogged by 'mucoid plaque' that results from cooking. Cooked starches and fats are major contributors to mucoid plaques.
- The body has to work hard to detoxify itself from the toxins that cooking produces.

About enzymes: separating the truth from fiction

One of the biggest arguments proponents of cooked food put forward against raw food is that we don't receive or need any enzyme from the food we eat. They say that the human body makes all its digestive enzymes. Nothing can be farther from the truth! Let us find out.

First, what are enzymes?

Enzymes are proteins manufactured by the pancreas (in the case of humans) _and_ all living organisms, including vegetables, fruits and animals. Yes. Even recently killed meat would have some active enzymes.

Enzymes help us digest the food we eat by:

- Rearranging the molecules of our food
- Synthesizing the chemicals of the food
- Adding elements to compounds
- Breaking down compounds

All this is done to help us extract the nutrients available in our foods.

Why is this processing required after we eat the food? Because many nutrients available in our foods are present in forms that our body would not be able to absorb without some processing of its own.

In humans, our pancreas is responsible for manufacturing our daily requirement of enzymes. Just like any other organ in the human body, the pancreas has a limited capacity. So, it can only produce so much of enzymes.

Do remember that it has other functions as well. Pancreas is also responsible for manufacturing the hormones that make us what we are and also secrete juices needed for many other important body functions like blood glucose balance, nerve functions, and many others.

If any food brings with it some enzymes necessary to digest it, our pancreas have to work less to digest and can concentrate on other tasks beneficial to our body.

By eating too much fast food or other hard to digest processed food, we place enormous pressure on our pancreas, and they start placing other important tasks in the backburner. In other words, our pancreas should be loaded with less digestive work so that they are able to work more on other important functions critical to our wellbeing.

Now where does all this fit into the raw food argument?

Bananas come with amylase, an enzyme that our pancreas also make to break down glucose. It converts the raw starch to sugar. Similarly, kiwis contain actinidin, another enzyme that helps digest kiwis. The same thing happens when we eat other easily digestible food, fruits, and vegetables as well.

The rules are really simple here. I am not asking you to understand any rocket science. *Anything that your body can easily digest is great for you!*

The lesson here is that raw foods are good not only for the wellbeing of our digestive systems but also for other vital systems of our bodies.

Chapter 2: The basic of a raw food diet

Diets are easy to start but extremely hard to sustain for long periods. They are also hard to maintain for busy people who are always on the move. So, if you have enough motivation to change your food habits, what will help you more than a 2-week diet is the awareness of what food is good for you and what is bad. This way, you can eat better in the long term.

Another problem with prescribing a specific diet is that the readers of this book may be spread across vast geographical areas, and the narrow guidelines of a diet might be a hurdle for them in terms of food availability. So, a set of broad guidelines would be best here.

Let us find out what type of food raw foodists should eat.

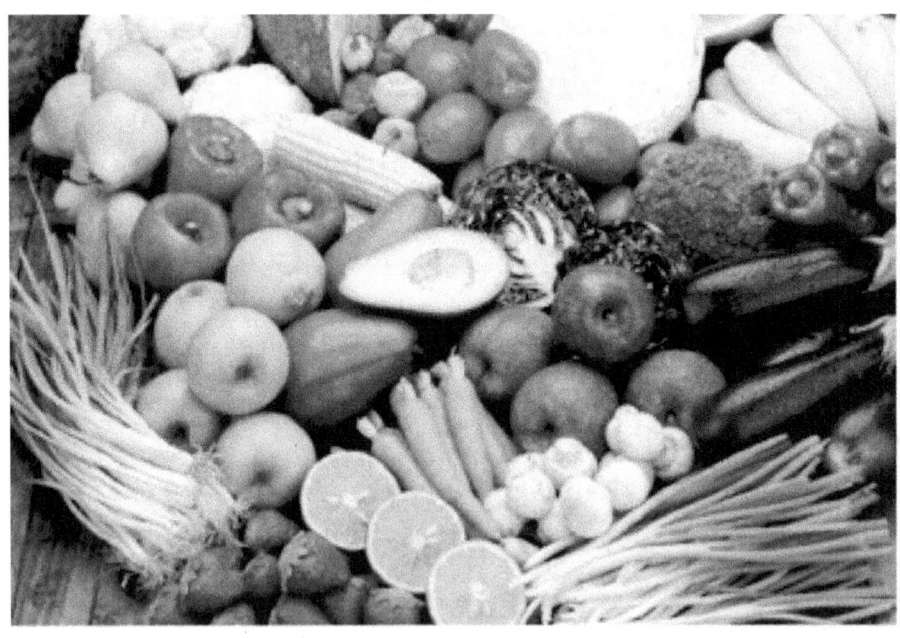

Speaking of fruits and vegetables, the first thing you should consider is which vegetables you should buy organic and which you should buy conventional (or non-organic). Generally, organic vegetables are costlier and harder to source but are always the healthier choice.

The guiding factor here should be pesticide load or the amount of pesticide used in growing those vegetables.

The following 12 fruits and vegetables are grown with the help of a huge amount of pesticides and you may consider getting the organic variety of them:

- ✓ Peaches
- ✓ Apples
- ✓ Sweet bell peppers
- ✓ Celery
- ✓ Nectarines
- ✓ Strawberries
- ✓ Cherries
- ✓ Lettuce
- ✓ Grapes (imported)
- ✓ Pears
- ✓ Spinach
- ✓ Potatoes

The following fruits and vegetables, on the other hand, have lowest traces of pesticides and can be had conventional (or non-organic):

- ✓ Broccoli
- ✓ Eggplant
- ✓ Cabbage
- ✓ Banana
- ✓ Kiwi
- ✓ Asparagus

- ✓ Sweet peas (frozen)
- ✓ Mango
- ✓ Pineapple
- ✓ Sweet corn (frozen)
- ✓ Avocado
- ✓ Onion

I hope this information would help you find food within your budget.

Juicing

Juicing your raw vegetables might sound like a chore, but you would be surprised at how easy it is with a proper food processor. It is easier than cooking, for sure. Since fruits are better tasting than vegetables, try to have fruits whole for your required fiber intake.

- More nutrients can be absorbed from vegetables by drinking them as juice.
- It is easier on your taste buds and your digestion system.
- Some vegetables taste horrible to chew. Juicing makes them more palatable, thus adding more variety (in terms of nutrition) to your food.

It is important to start by juicing vegetables you enjoy. It helps you continue for long.

Also, listen to your body. There might be some vegetables that might not be able to digest as smoothly as others. I find it troublesome to drink (juiced) cabbage in one go, but I do fine when I spread it out and have it in two or three installments over the day.

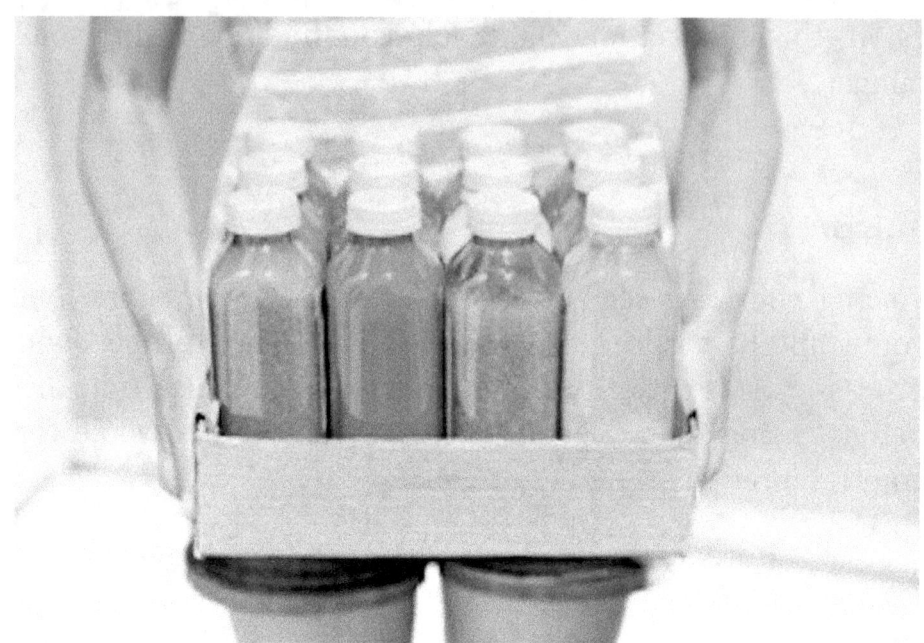

As far as eating raw vegetables is concerned, there are some vegetables that are healthier than others and provide more nutrients. The following vegetables are more healthful when eaten raw:

- Asparagus
- Avocado (actually a fruit)
- Beet greens
- Bok Choy
- Broccoli
- Brussels sprouts
- Cauliflower
- Celery
- Chicory
- Chinese cabbage
- Chives
- Collard greens

- Cucumbers
- Dandelion greens
- Endive
- Escarole
- Fennel
- Green and red cabbage
- Kale
- Kohlrabi
- Lettuce: romaine, red leaf, green leaf
- Mustard greens

- Onions
- Parsley
- Peppers: red, green, yellow and hot
- Tomatoes
- Turnips
- Spinach
- Zucchini
- Beets
- Eggplant
- Jicama
- Winter squash

Fermented foods

When (some) vegetables are fermented, they become doubly nutritious. The good enzymes already present in the vegetables tend to flourish when fermented. The process of fermentation pre-digests the starch content of a food and makes it easier for your body to process them.

- Create an environment full of minerals, probiotic and enzymes that help us digest food.
- They fill your guts with substances like lactobacilli, which help us keep our system clean.
- Fermented food also helps detoxify our systems.

As an added bonus, fermented food also helps you control your cravings for sweets!

Some examples of fermented foods are sauerkraut and kimchee, both easily available in stores. There are many other vegetables you can buy fermented, and some vegetables like cabbage, carrots, beets, etc. you can ferment yourself. You can also eat curd tofu and other milk-derived fermented foods.

One word of caution here: In case you are getting fermented food off the rack from stores, please make sure they are not salted and pasteurized. These two processes totally defeat the purpose behind eating food raw.

Chapter 3: Some guidelines for following raw food diets

Some vegetables when eaten raw can be harmful to you in many different ways. I have mentioned some of them and also given the reason behind my advice. However, the best advice I could give you regarding what to eat and what not to eat is simple:

Consult a dietician before you start.

You don't want to end up flat on your bed with some deadly condition. Some general tips are mentioned below.

Besides fruits and vegetables, you can include various nuts and seeds in your diet such as almonds, cashews, Brazil nuts, hazelnuts, pine nuts, pumpkin seeds, flax seeds, sunflower seeds, etc. Grains can also find their place in a raw food diet, and you can have them whole, soaked or sprouted. As a raw foodist, you can enjoy a variety of these – rice, wheat, oats, quinoa, barley, rye, buckwheat. When it comes to oil, you can use any unprocessed or cold-processed oils such as palm oil, coconut oil, and olive oil. If you want to add sweeteners to your desserts, you can add raw agave nectar, raw honey, and unprocessed maple syrup.

Vegetables to avoid

One vegetable that should generally be avoided raw, for reasons obvious to all of my readers, is the potato. I don't think anyone ever enjoyed raw potato. Also, raw potatoes carry a toxic compound called solanine.

Uncooked or even undercooked beans carry a substance called glycoprotein lectin, which is toxic to us humans. According to the US FDA, as little as 5 raw kidney beans can be a cause for trouble. Castor beans can also cause these same problems.

Raw broccoli, cabbage, cauliflower and other cruciferous vegetables are fine for most, but some experience gas and bloating. The culprits here are some sugars typical to cruciferous vegetables in raw condition. Also, those with thyroid and related conditions should avoid raw cruciferous vegetables as well because they contain thyroid inhibitors and can worsen thyroid if already present.

Bitter almonds, more common in Europe than America, can be dangerous when had raw. They contain high amounts of hydrogen cyanide, which can cause vomiting, headache, and convulsions. In extreme cases, hydrogen cyanide causes breathing problems, too. The same is the case with cassava, chaya, and tapioca.

Olives taste bitter and should be had only when cooked or as olive oil. Wild mushrooms are a source of many allergies as well.

There are many other vegetables (especially those local vegetables) that may be toxic for raw human consumption, and it is impossible to put up an exhaustive list here. That is the reason I have suggested a consultation with a dietician before you embark on a raw food adventure.

Chapter 4: Mistakes in a raw food diet

If you have started following a raw food diet, chances are that in the beginning you will feel weak or suffer crises, which may lead you to doubt the benefits of this diet. You should know that this is all normal because your body needs some time to adapt to this process of cleaning itself from all the accumulated garbage and toxins. You may experience this kind of discomfort even if you are an experienced raw foodist. Then, this may be a signal that your body doesn't get the necessary vitamins or other nutrients, probably because the range of food you eat is not wide.

- **Don't forget to eat greens**

This discomfort that you may feel in the beginning will quickly disappear once you start eating enough greens. To avoid this kind of trouble, try including enough greens in your soups and smoothies.

- **Don't jump into it straight away**

Although raw food is really powerful at cleansing your body, you can bet that your body won't like it. It will need some time to adapt to this new diet. So, you should reduce the cooked foods gradually so that your body processes will stay regular, and your body will have time to adapt. Otherwise, you will experience certain discomforts such as bloating, digestion problems, chills, and headaches.

- **Not eating enough**

Raw food is not only about fruits and vegetables. They are great, but they are not enough to support your body with the necessary fuel. Instead, you will need to rely on some denser sources of protein and make sure not to forget fats. So, you should also enjoy various nuts and seeds, coconut and avocado. These are all high-calorie foods that your body needs to work properly.

- **Take it easy on nuts and fruits**

Although fruits and nuts make a great combination, you should know when to stop. Since fruits are great sources of sugar, and nuts are rich in fats, there is a great possibility that you will have some digestive problems and will gain some weight if you overdo nuts and fruits. So, bear in mind that you should eat fruits when your stomach is empty so as not to put a strain on digestion, and don't rely on nuts as the only source of protein. Raw grains, greens and seeds are also rich in proteins, so they should be included in your raw food diet as well.

- **Don't get crazy**

Following a raw food diet doesn't mean that you should fear cooked food. If, for instance, there are vegetables that you can't digest, then you can boil them and allow your body to digest them and absorb their nutrients. Also, some foods contain more nutrients when they are cooked. So, it is fine if you occasionally eat some cooked meal.

Like any other diet, a raw food diet should also be balanced. Listen to your body and find what suits it best.

Chapter 5: How I fell in love with raw food

You may say that you eat vegetables in your salads, but you have to admit that you don't eat large portions of salads and these are mainly made with two or three different vegetables. What if you have a salad with six different vegetables? You will have a bowl rich in essential minerals, vitamins and antioxidants.

When I first thought about a raw food diet, I was fascinated by all those vibrant and lively colors. Also, I discovered a whole variety of foods that I hadn't used before. I decided to give it a try and see how my body will react to it, as I wanted something that will clean my body because it really needed a change, and it deserved to finally be treated right.

I started slowly, as I was scared that my body won't accept the change well. So, first I tried to substitute one cooked meal with a raw food meal. After some time, I had only one cooked meal a day and I realized how good I feel. Finally, I turned to a raw food diet completely, and the changes I noticed were amazing.

It may sound strange, but I noticed some spiritual change happening inside me. It was like my mind opened up now that it was not fogged with all the garbage from processed food. I felt lighter and my intuition improved. Thus, I started noticing all the small things around me that I hadn't noticed before.

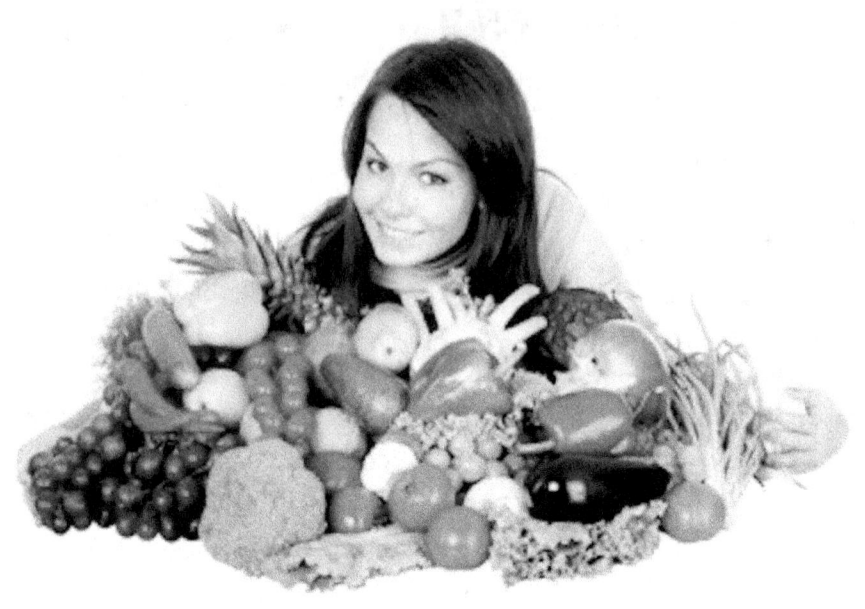

What is even more, my digestion improved, and I also dropped a few extra pounds and now look perfectly slim. The reason behind this is that raw food has higher water content than processed food, and because of that you eat less and feel fuller.

By eating raw food, I also know that my teeth and gums have enough workout to stay healthy. Namely, raw food requires you to chew more and this stimulates blood to come to these parts of your mouth.

Raw food has done a world of good for my skin as well. There's an explanation for that as well. Certain raw foods, such as tomatoes and carrots, contain beta-carotene. When you eat these foods raw, you supply your body with high amounts of beta-carotene, which is converted into vitamin A when digested, and it is responsible for building collagen and stimulating your skin cells to grow. All this makes my skin elastic, young and silky, and I don't even have to use any skincare products.

Now I feel I'm bursting with energy and am definitely more focused. This is probably because cooked food takes longer to digest, and those partially digested carbohydrates, proteins, and fats tend to clog up my arteries and digestive system.

Soon enough after turning to raw food, I discovered that I can still eat delicious meals and stay healthy and young, and this eventually improved my life. So, I think now it's pretty clear why I fell in love with raw food. I hope you will share this passion with me.

Conclusion

This book is my attempt to tell a story about falling in love with raw food. You will learn about the reasons that made me turn to this kind of diet and all the benefits that all of you may experience if you follow my example. I hope that you will soon embark on this adventure and start thinking about raw food the same way I do.

About the Author

Anastasia Schultz is a woman interested in everything that can bring vitality to her life. As a mother of two sons, she finds a great pleasure in discovering the powers of food in order to keep her family healthy. Her many friends and relatives, some of whom are doctors and professors, are another valuable source where she can learn how to use food to stay healthy. Because of everything she has discovered so far, she supports the power of raw food.

Her tendency to help others inspires her to write about her discoveries and share all the valuable information she has on improving one's health and life through food. As she believes that small steps can lead to big changes, she hopes that this book will help her readers find the answers to all the questions they may have about a raw vegan diet.